Cognitive Behavioral Therapy: Heal Your Life!

5 Powerful Steps to Overcome Anxiety, Negative Emotions & Depression

By Maya Faro

Copyright Maya Faro©2016

Maya Faro© Copyright 2016 - All rights reserved.

Legal Notice:

This book is copyright protected. It for personal use only.

Disclaimer Notice:

Please note the information contained in this document is for educational and entertainment purposes only. Every attempt has been made to provide accurate, up to date and completely reliable information. No warranties of any kind are expressed or implied.

Readers acknowledge that the author is not engaging in the rendering of legal, financial, medical or professional advice. By reading this document, the reader agrees that under no circumstances are we responsible for any losses, direct or indirect, which are incurred as a result of the use of information contained within this document, including, but not limited to, errors, omissions, or inaccuracies.

Contents

Letter from the Author 9

Chapter 1 – Step 1 – Understanding That Anxiety Is Trying to Be Your Friend 14

    There is a Point to Anxiety 14

        Anxiety - American Psychological Association 15

    Anxiety Is an Emotion: A Whole Body Experience 16

    Some Triggers You May Not Have Thought Of 17

    The Function of Emotions 19

    CBT Activity 21

Chapter 2 – Step 2: Let's See How Anxious You Are and Plot A Course To Being As Anxious As You Choose To Be! 26

    CBT Activity: SYMPTOMS CHECKLIST 26

Chapter 3 – Step 3: What Is Causing Your Anxious Response? 32

    Understanding Cognitive Behavioral Approaches and Finding Out What Your Unconscious Beliefs Are 32

    CBT Definition 32

        In-Depth: Cognitive Behavioral Therapy | Psych Central 33

    CBT Activity 34

Chapter 4 – Step 4. Learn the Thinking Styles Which Make You Most Anxious and Turn Them Around 43

    STYLES OF THINKING 43

    Putting up a Filter 45

    CBT Activity 47

    Black and White Thinking 47

    If It Applied Once, It Will Apply to Everything 48

    CBT Activity 49

I Can Read Your Mind 50
CBT Activity... 51
Something Terrible Will Happen... 52
CBT Activity... 52
They Must Have Meant Me 52
CBT Activity... 53
I Should.... 53
CBT Activity... 55
SUMMARY 55
MAKE A RATIONAL COMEBACK AND GIVE YOURSELF 'PERMISSION.' 56

Chapter 5 – Step 5: From Anxious to Assured. The Transformation 65
INCREASING YOUR POSITIVE EMOTIONS........................ 65
DAILY POSITIVE EXPERIENCES 69
CBT Activity... 70

Chapter 6 - Living an Anxiety-Free, Assured Life.................... 71
Another Step to Try Out If This Feels Right for You 71
The Skills of Mindfulness.. 71
When You Feel Happy 73
When You Feel Anxiety... 73

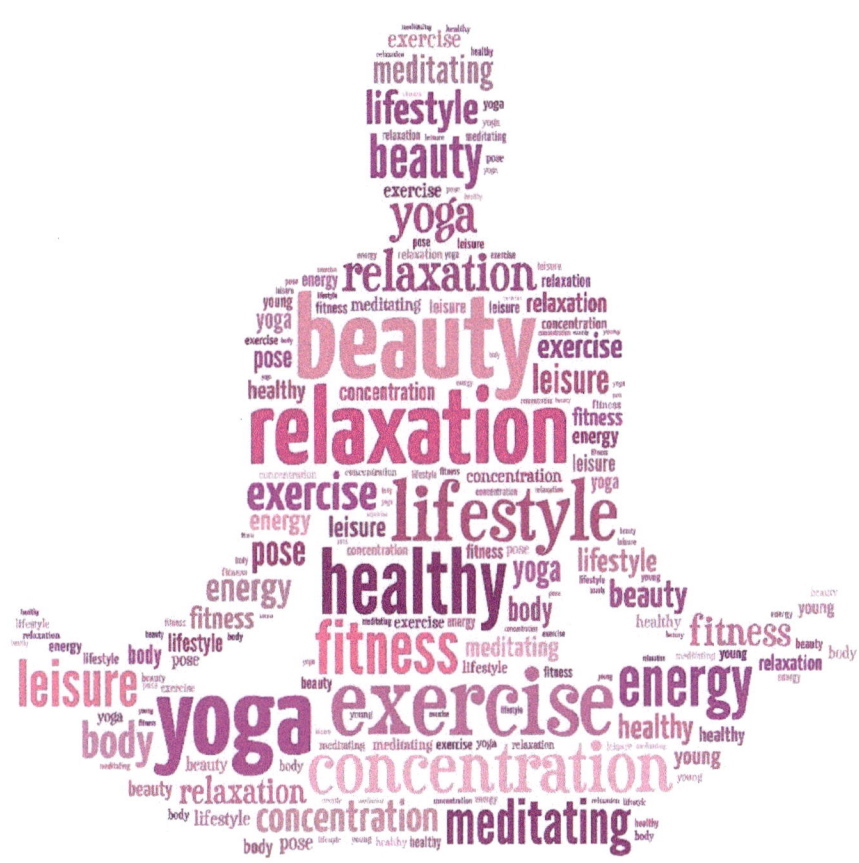

Letter from the Author

Anxiety is a tough emotion to feel on a regular basis. I know personally just how it can cripple you. Freezing into immobility, unable to go forward to grab opportunities, take a chance or even be a bit optimistic, because of being so scared and worried by 'what might be'. Almost everyone has a degree of anxiety in their life but, although it is uncomfortable when it arises, it is bearable, and they do move on. But for others, it takes its toll on their health, happiness, and joy in life.

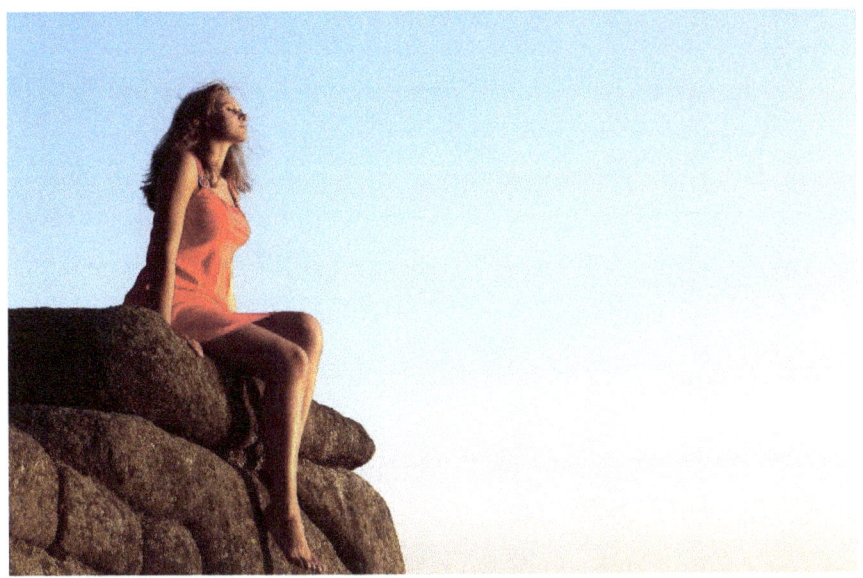

That is why I am writing this book. My mother was one such person. From a happy, exuberant child she slowly morphed into a frightened, over anxious woman who didn't dare to do anything too risky – and for her, most actions were risky! I could see she had a far less happy life than she deserved and I determined never to be like that. However, some of the patterns are learnt and there were periods in my life when anxiety attacks were the norm and it took courage and a lot of awareness to change that. I learnt great deal and began to help others who were suffering through a mixture of anxiety, guilt, shame and worry and they began to change too.

For all of us an important aspect was to learn that anxiety is trying to be your friend. But, as with friends in your life, you don't have to live with them! The secret is not to let it run your life. And certainly not to let it ruin your life.

Anxiety is a bit different for everyone. Different things trigger each of us. Different thoughts, beliefs and memories play a part. What is common however is a Vicious Circle of events which is where we will focus. These events are unhelpful beliefs which swing into action when an outside situation reminds you unconsciously of something that has bothered you in the past. These beliefs then trigger off unhelpful emotions (fear, anxiety, worry, anger, agitation) which are all too familiar and make it hard to think logically about the situation. These emotions then kick-start a series of unhelpful actions, which lead us back round to feeling bad, sad or mad! And anxious!

What you will do in this book is learn how to turn these Vicious Circles into Virtuous Circles.

Virtuous Circles leave you feeling better about yourself, other people and life. The secret tool is your self-talk. We have negative thinking styles which become the way we talk to ourselves and those thinking styles are right at the heart of our anxiety. The second secret tool is 'self-soothing'. Self-soothing skills are also right at the heart of managing Anxiety. And you will learn just how to develop these skills right here.

In my own learning, I also found the cognitive behavioral approach gave me a very structured way to work with the Vicious Circle of emotions, thoughts, and actions. It worked well for me and the clients I had and when we began to build on the Cognitive Behavioral structure by developing our self-soothing skills life became transformed.

This book is the result of all our learning, hard work (yes, I am being honest, it took blood, sweat and tears to get those Circles spinning the other way) and successes. The good news is that it can be done; it is being done right now by brave people who want to change. Or sometimes they aren't brave, they are just desperate because they don't want another year, another decade… like the last ones where constant, daily struggles and anxiety beset them. Is that you?

Do you want to change?

It's a very important question because many of us say we want to change but when the steps are in front of us we find that we struggle because deep down, we don't really think we can do it. However, I think you DO want to change because you have read this far.

Take a step by step approach, don't rush and above all have compassion for yourself as you gently explore this aspect of you. Smile softly and remind yourself that you have the right to help yourself experience a happy, assured, low stress life and that you believe change is possible. Because it is! And most especially it is true of you!

Stick with me, do the activities, keep a journal, practice and…..if you would find it easier to do with another person, find a counsellor who will support you as you change from Anxious to Assured and transform your life.

Enjoy the journey. I'm right there with you.

Maya Faro

Chapter 1 – Step 1 – Understanding That Anxiety Is Trying to Be Your Friend

There is a Point to Anxiety

Anxiety has a bad rap! It's uncomfortable to feel. It is linked with other emotions such as fear, uncertainty, and apprehension. It makes blood pressure rise because our bodies get ready for fight or flight in the face of an imagined outcome. It gets in the way of happy times. All in all, it is an emotion that takes the WOW factor out of life as we keep bringing ourself down to earth with a huge bump as we worry about one thing after another.

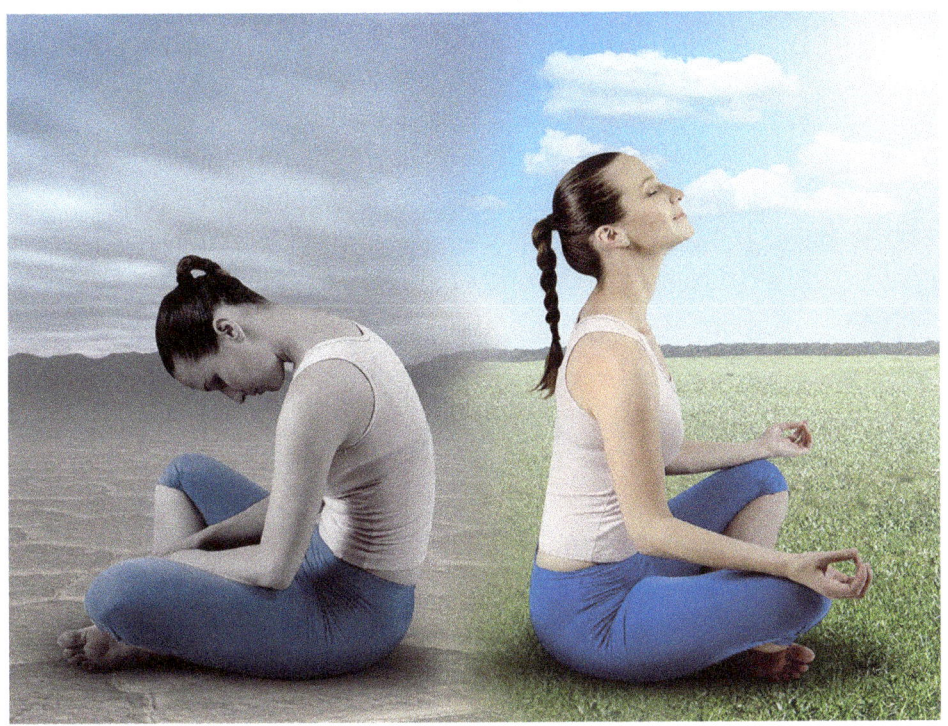

So what exactly is it?

In a nutshell:

"**Anxiety** is an emotion characterized by feelings of tension, worried thoughts and physical changes like increased blood pressure. People with **anxiety** disorders usually have recurring intrusive thoughts or concerns. They may avoid certain situations out of worry."

Anxiety - American Psychological Association
www.apa.org/topics/**anxiety**/

Anxiety Is an Emotion: A Whole Body Experience

The first thing to know about it is that it is an emotion. What we need to know about emotions are that they are 'whole body' experiences. This means they consist of thoughts, feelings, sensations and behaviors. Thoughts, beliefs, old patterns of reacting, a mixture of feelings including fear, guilt, shame and worry begin to course through the nervous system and trigger off the start of a bout of anxiety. This may end in an avoidance of whatever started the emotional response. At worst it can end in an anxiety attack and a reinforcement of a phobic response to similar triggers.

Anyone who has experienced an anxiety attack will know that this is a frightening experience. You get disorientated, breathless, panic overwhelms you, and it is very hard to return to a more balanced body state. It helps to know that the oxygen/carbon dioxide levels in your body go out of whack and breathing into a paper bag can bring your blood chemistry back to normal and your brain will return to being able to think again. It's definitely not something we want to happen – and having had one attack there is a secret fear left behind that it will happen again. This of course, further reinforces the avoidance of whatever set off the initial emotion of anxiety. It's one of those horrible Vicious Circles I spoke about in the Introduction, and we have to find ways to turn that into a Virtuous Circle, step by step.

But before we look at you and your anxiety patterns in more depth have a think about the following.

Some Triggers You May Not Have Thought Of

I once had a client come to me about their intense bouts of anxiety and how they had recently had a panic attack while on the local station. This poor person was terribly upset and frightened by how out of control they had felt. As we discussed the situation and the triggers it emerged that they drank 10 cups of coffee per day before going home from the office at night.

I asked them to cut out the coffee (and tea) for a week before we started doing any other exploration of their 'anxiety syndrome.' They did this – even though they weren't keen on the herbal alternatives! That change completely stopped their sense of apprehension and 'jitters'. They had been reading their body's reaction to caffeine and calling it anxiety because that was what all the physical symptoms felt like. But in fact, it was mainly chemical!

The following checklist may also help you to know that there is a pile of things that increase feelings of anxiety which you may be doing and making the anxiety worse for yourself.

Mark all that apply to you, then add others you may be aware of, but that aren't on the list. By building awareness of how you make yourself more sensitive can help you reduce, or even banish, feelings of anxiety like the client above:

- Too much or too little sleep
- Too much junk food
- Dehydration
- Too much caffeine

- Hunger and poor nutrition
- Overeating or under eating
- Injuries or wounds
- Physical illness
- Financial problems
- Underemployment or unemployment
- Overworking
- Eating too much sugar
- Eating too much fat
- Recent losses or accidents
- Recent natural disasters or social horrors such as mass shootings
- Current relationship difficulties
- Being a victim of crime (assault, rape, theft, etc.)
- Lack of exercise
- Tendency to dwelling on a recent personal failure
- Other_____

All of these things increase your reactions and make you more impulsive, super emotional and bring about a state of emotional anxious suffering. Even if you are a typically cool, calm and collected person you will get overly emotional when you are tired, easily slipping into irritability and anxiety. The antidote?

Well, in this case, it's sleep. But also be aware that if you've been amping up on coffee all day, you will be more likely to fidget and feel like you are really nervous about something – but not be able to put your finger on what it is you are anxious about.

Can you recognise some of the ways you make it harder for yourself and think about how to cut down on them.

That was just a quick activity to get you into the swing of observing yourself and making the links between your behaviour, thoughts, feelings and your body. You'll be doing more of that as we go through the book. Now let's have a look at emotions and why on earth we have these, often pesky, but always needed, things! In other words, how are emotions like anxiety our friends?

The Function of Emotions

1. Emotions prompt and organize us for action:

When a particular emotion is triggered, your whole body goes on alert so that it is ready for fighting, fleeing or freezing in reaction to the threat. Anger can organize you mentally and physiologically to become aggressive. Fear will get you ready to flee, if necessary; your mind begins fear-related thoughts, and your body is primed to run for safety. Your entire biological makeup is primed to take action consistent with whatever emotion has been triggered. This is why we are such holistic beings. You can't separate mind, emotions and body.

2. Emotions give us valuable information about what is going on in any particular situation:

Emotions are like a motion-detecting or warning system telling us that something is happening in our environment that we should know about. This warning system can alert us to physical danger, or give us information about how a social interaction is going. It is important to be aware of your emotions so that you can hear what they are telling you because they can alert you to a threat, a discomfort or give you a thumbs up that a situation is benign and supportive. Paying attention to what your emotions are telling you can make a difference to your safety or assist you with improving relationships and enjoying life more. In both cases, emotions may tell you that you need to change your behavior to become more effective at meeting your needs or at forging quality relationships.

3. Emotions are for motivating us:

To return to the very word itself, "motion," emotions get you going to do things. These may be work, relationships, or seeking food or more pleasure. Strong emotions can help you in overcoming obstacles between you and something you want. Jealousy may motivate you to protect a relationship by being more attentive to your partner. Anger may lead you to stand up for your rights when you are being mistreated. Anxiety will motivate you to protect yourself. This is really important when it comes to managing your anxiety and starting to soothe yourself.

4. Emotions are fundamentally our friends. Every single one of them!

All that has been said above is summed up in this statement. Emotions are inherently, essentially, and fundamentally adaptive. That is, your emotions are friends and helpers. Sometimes I liken emotions to shepherds that try to guide us to safety and well-being. Even painful emotions such as fear or anxiety can guide us away from danger. Interest can help us to expand our learning and self-mastery through learning.

If you have written off your emotions because you sometimes find yourself being too emotional and over-whelmed, it is time to change your mind. It is time to appreciate the natural functions and advantages of emotions and start listening to them for their words of wisdom. Then learn to step back and use your power of reasoning too so that the actions you end up taking will be a careful blend of emotional information and logical information.

So as far as your feelings of anxiety are concerned the way into this is to begin to unpick the thoughts and beliefs that underlie you feeling of fear and apprehension. Remember the Vicious Circle - although we may not be aware of it, our unconscious thoughts and beliefs trigger our feeling state. Now we are going to start being more conscious of emotions, then thoughts, then actions... This is an exciting journey.

CBT Activity

Reflect on the ebb and flow of your anxiety:

You will see that your emotions vary in how strong they feel. One moment you can be terribly anxious and only moments later feel a little bit worried.

ANXIETY

Think of a time when you were so anxious that all you wanted to do was hide, withdraw, avoid others, panic, or freak out. Think about your most anxious moment, whatever that might be for you. Fill in the following:

Situation:_____
_____

_____
_____

Your thoughts about the situation (how did you interpret it?)_____

_____
_____

Intensity of your anxiety (0-100)_____

Describe what happened after you felt that way (were things the same, made worse, made better?)_____
_____

How long did it take you to get back to your normal mood?

    Seconds (how many)_____

    Minutes (how many)_____

    Hours (how many)_____

    A day or more (how many)_____

When you relaxed, what was the strength of your anxiety (0-100?)_____

Now what?

You see how emotions vary in intensity; they flow in and out of being and that often time passing makes a difference. In other words what you have discovered is that emotions are biochemical states in our bodies, and the chemistry needs a bit of time to come back into balance again. Now it is time to explore how anxious you are and get down to working through a self-help plan, step by step.

But before you do that here's something lovely you may start experimenting with now. It's the concept of self-soothing. Usually, it is our self-talk that creates states of anxiety. It certainly perpetuates them. You are going to learn more about that self-talk and how to make it work positively for you but first, let's just gently start bringing in some self-soothing practices to your life as an antidote to that overload of anxiety adrenaline you carry around.

Activity

SELF-SOOTHING ACTIVITIES TO BEGIN TRYING OUT RIGHT NOW

Remember, when you are anxious you are frightened, worried, and your body is prepared for fighting, fleeing or freezing up as ways to protect yourself. Just like a child who has got into a bit of a state because she/he can't work out a way to deal with it, your body needs to be soothed so it can begin to come out of that Reaction Response and into the Relaxation Response. People have many ways to soothe themselves. Start experimenting with one of the following – choose the one that appeals to you most. The easiest way is to start with the senses.

Vision

- Hang pictures on your walls
- Take an art book out of the library
- Buy a decorative centrepiece
- Put up seasonal decorations
- Look at trees, grass, plants, rivers, ponds, fountains or the sea

Hearing

- Listen to classical music
- Listen to mellow instrumental music
- Buy one of those meditation CD's with nature sounds and relax to it

- Play a musical instrument
- Sing to yourself

Smell

- Burn incense or scented candles
- Go to a bakery, stand around and take in the smells
- Rub scented oil or lotion over your body
- Bake bread or brownies

Touch

- Get a massage
- Hug someone, or hug a tree
- Go for a swim
- Take a long, luxurious bath, or a long hot shower
- Rub oil all over your body
- Put clean sheets on your bed and climb in just luxuriating in the feel of it
- Put on silk pyjamas
- Stand in the wind and feel how it blows over your body and face

Taste

- Slowly eat your favourite food, savouring every bite
- Slowly drink a warm drink, like milk or chocolate milk, feeling its warmth entering your body
- Eat hot toast
- Eat peppermint or cinnamon sweets slowly

Keep this self-soothing idea in your mind and now …..

Next chapter, please...

Chapter 2 – Step 2: Let's See How Anxious You Are and Plot A Course To Being As Anxious As You Choose To Be!

Let's get right down to it....

CBT Activity: SYMPTOMS CHECKLIST

Use This Checklist to help you stop anxiety running your life. We need to start somewhere specific (it's just easier that way!). So complete the following checklist, to get clearer about your symptoms, your triggers, and their intensity.

Rate your symptoms below for the degree of discomfort they cause you, using the following a 10-point scale:

Slight discomfort   Moderate discomfort   Extreme discomfort

1   2   3   4   5   6   7   8   9   10

SYMPTOM (Disregard those you don't experience)	*Degree of Discomfort (1-10) Now*	*Level of Discomfort (1-10) after working through the Cognitive Behavioral Approach*

		(you'll come back to this)

Anxiety in specific situations

- *Tests*
- *Deadlines*
- *Interviews*
- *Other:*

Anxiety in personal relationships

- *Spouse*
- *Parents*
- *Children*
- *Other:*

Anxiety, general – regardless of the situation or the people involved

Typical feelings you have when you are anxious

Depressed

Hopeless

Powerless

Self-Esteem low – no sense of worth

Hostility increases generally (start blaming others or yourself very harshly)

Anger towards someone increases

Irritability generally increases (very hard to settle and be warm to others)

Resentment gets stronger

Phobias increase in intensity– specify object or situation that gets worse – spiders, being out of the house, meeting new people...

Obsessions, unwanted thoughts... increase. Can't stop going over and over conversations in your head trying to work out a meaning/say what you wish you'd said

Muscular tension gets worse

Procrastination increases

Overeating takes place more often

Smoking increases

Problem-drinking gets worse

Gambling increases

Overspending increases

Physical pain/illness gets worse

Compulsions, checking things many times... getting more frequent

Insomnia increasing

Sleeping difficulties on many nights

Unwanted sexual fantasies increasing

Unwanted sexual behaviour increasing

Perfectionism gets more pronouncing

Ineffective problem-solving

The checklist includes things that may not be associated with your anxious state – but they are all behaviors or states that are commonly linked to being anxious.

Note which ones are your top 5.

_____

_____

_____

_____

_____

And which ones are your bottom 3?

_____

_____

_____

NB:(Symptoms you don't have aren't scored at all so they are not in the bottom three. We are only looking at the ones where you scored yourself as having some kind of discomfort.)

Now, contrary to what you might be expecting, you need to choose the highest score in your bottom three! This is the one you are going to explore and change first.

It always works better if you begin with something that is easier to 'move' then when you feel successful and have confidence in the system move to the symptom which is the bottom score of the top five. Then work with that. Only after that do you start to work with the top three?

Please don't be tempted to jump in and tackle the toughest challenges – remember. Compassion for Yourself!

This is a good time to congratulate yourself because it takes courage to face your anxiety and begin to look at it long enough to see if there are any patterns in its appearance – or disappearance – or continual appearance! To acknowledge that you feel anxious most, or all, of the time, is a big step. But, with compassion for yourself and a growing recognition that all your emotions are there to communicate something important to you-you can move onto the next chapter and start to unpick the thoughts and beliefs you hold which are complicating your anxious state. This is step three where we use the cognitive behavioral approach to help us move on.

Chapter 3 –Step 3: What Is Causing Your Anxious Response?

Understanding Cognitive Behavioral Approaches and Finding Out What Your Unconscious Beliefs Are

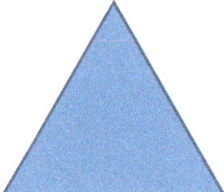

Feelings

Thoughts **Behaviors**

Cognitive behavioural approaches think of a person as being a 'whole unit,' made up of thoughts and feelings and behaviors all taking place within a body. In fact, they say that the unconscious thoughts and beliefs (beliefs are a set of fixed thoughts) we have, drive our feeling responses and those trigger us to behave in certain set ways and that those set ways bring about biochemical states in our body. All the different components feed, reinforce and escalate each other so it isn't surprising that we feel overwhelmed with anxiety when it gets going. This is another way of describing the Vicious Circle we talked about earlier.

CBT Definition

Cognitive behavioral therapy (CBT) is a short-term, goal-oriented psychotherapy **treatment** that takes a hands-on, practical approach to problem-solving. Its goal is to change patterns of thinking or **behavior** that are behind people's difficulties, and so change the way they feel.Feb 22, 2007

[In-Depth: Cognitive Behavioral Therapy | Psych Central](#)
*psychcentral.com/lib/in-depth-**cognitive-behavioral-therapy**/*

So the thing to take from this very short overview of cognitive behavioural approaches is that the psychologists believe that:

- by understanding how we trigger ourselves into an anxiety state though our beliefs and thoughts

- and also understanding more about the feelings that rush upon us at this point

- we can then learn alternative ways to talk to ourselves and soothe ourselves

- and so we can begin to control our anxiety.

Let's take that bit by bit

AUTOMATIC THOUGHTS/BELIEFS AFFECT EMOTION

Here are some examples of our unconscious belief patterns that can trigger off the overwhelm of anxiety. Notice how charged some of them are. We can organise the unhelpful thoughts and beliefs into three categories: demands we place on ourselves about:

- ourself,
- other people,

- the world/life.

CBT Activity

Looking at the three kinds of demands below, do any ring true for you? If so, mark those statements that reflect your own automatic thoughts, then use the blank lines below to list any of your other unique automatic thoughts.

1. <u>Your demands on yourself</u>

Mark the demands that you identify with and then rate the strength with which you hold this belief (0 = not at all, 100 = hugely!):

- ☐ *I must do well in everything I put my hand to, and if I don't, it's awful   Intensity _____*
- ☐ *I must be approved of by all the important people in my life, and if I don't, it's awful*
       Intensity _____
- ☐ *I'm not lovable if I fail at an important task*
       Intensity _____
- ☐ *I've got no value/worthless if I'm not loved and don't do well at things*
       Intensity _____
- ☐ *Everyone will hate me if I am not great at everything I do*
       Intensity _____
- ☐ *I have to do everything quickly so that everyone is pleased with me*
       Intensity _____
- ☐ *I must please everybody/the important people in my life*
       Intensity _____
- ☐ *I must always try hard at everything I do*

    Intensity _____
- [ ] *I must be tough and never show my emotions*
    Intensity
*Other:*_____

_____

<u>*Your demands about other people*</u>
- [ ] *Others should treat me justly and fairly*
    Intensity _____
- [ ] *Others must treat me with respect*
    Intensity _____
- [ ] *When others treat me poorly, they deserve to be punished*
    Intensity _____
- [ ] *When others don't give me what I want, they must pay for it in some way*
    Intensity _____
- [ ] *If people do what they shouldn't, then they're bad people*
    Intensity _____
- [ ] *I never like people who let me down*
    Intensity _____
- [ ] *It feels like a disaster when I don't get what I want from other people*
    Intensity _____
- [ ] *Other:*_____

_____

2. <u>*Your demands about the world or life conditions*</u>
- [ ] *I have to have a life that is easy and comfortable*
    Intensity _____
- [ ] *I can't stand too many challenges in life, but life always throws one challenge after the other at me*
    Intensity _____
- [ ] *There should never be any pain*

Intensity _____
- ☐ *Life should be fair*
    Intensity _____
- ☐ *If I'm good, the world (or God, or the universe) should treat me well   Intensity* _____
- ☐ *Other:*_____
_____

Finally, put on your thinking cap and try to come up with at least one challenge to each of the thoughts you have marked. Just ask yourself "is this true?"

For example:

☐ *I must do well in everything I put my hand to, and if I don't, it's awful*	*Is this true?*
	Your thoughts?
	<u>*A New Perspective on your Beliefs:*</u>
	There are many things to be done in life so doing everything perfectly is unrealistic.
☐ *I must be approved of by all the important people in my life, and if I don't, it's awful*	*Is this true?*
	Your thoughts?
	<u>*A New Perspective on your Beliefs*</u>

People are so different and want such different things from you that you could never please or get approval from everyone! Think about what you want and approve of yourself for being your own person.

☐ *I never like people who let me down*

Is this true?

Your thoughts?

<u>A New Perspective on your Beliefs</u>

You can stand back from a situation and see if the other person may have had another reason for their action which was nothing to do with you.

☐ *It feels like a disaster when I don't get what I want from other people*

Is this true?

Your thoughts?

A New Perspective on your Beliefs

You can step back and see what happened from a more distant perspective. It often changes things when you do that.

☐ Life should be fair

Is this true?

Your thoughts?

A New Perspective on your Beliefs

You can be disappointed if something doesn't work out 'fairly' but it wastes your good energy if you rail against life as life will always win. Practice "letting go" of that expectation

- ☐ *If I'm good, the world (or God, or the universe) should treat me well*

Is this true?

Your thoughts?

<u>*A New Perspective on your Beliefs*</u>
You can treat yourself well no matter what life is throwing at you.

It can be helpful if you experiment with a Thoughts Diary for a week or even a few days. That way you can unpack some of those 'quick as lightning' thoughts that flash through you and become part of the trigger for being anxious. See below:

THOUGHTS & BELIEFS DIARY

To begin to get to know how powerful your unconscious thoughts are, and what role they play in your anxious feelings and behavior, try making your own thoughts diary. Make a note each time you experience anxiety. Include everything you tell yourself to keep the emotion going. One of my clients made these notes on a day in her week.

For example:

08:15-Anxiety and anger-Stuck in traffic-Late...-The boss will be angry...-I'll be the last one in and then I'll never catch up all day...-I must be punctual

-Once something goes wrong it gets worse

How true now- 90% How true later-40%

10:30-Anxiety-Given additional work-I'll be here all night... can't stand it again.... kids will struggle with homework if I'm late-I've got to do my duty- 100%-30%

11:50-Anxiety-Computer breaks down-I'll never get it done now...Oh God...I should work faster, or he'll get angry-I have to be perfect worker-100%-55%

12:30-Anxiety-Have to work through lunch-My stomach is really going to hurt...- I can't bear it, and I'll get a headache-I have to do my duty and be perfect!-80%-20%

04:00-Anger-More work comes in-Why don't these jerks get enough help... -This is too much for one person I always get dumped on-People take advantage of me-100%-60%

05:00-Anxiety-Working late-have to call partner-He's going to blow his stack now this has happened again....-I have to be a perfect partner-100%-0%

06:45-Depression-Driving home-This is my whole life.... -There's no way out of this-Life is hard for me-100%-35%

These are all typical examples of situations that arise in everyday life which can be part of a trigger to feeling anxious. However, you may also notice a few thoughts and beliefs you have about the emotions you are having as a result of your first thoughts! We get pretty complicated as humans!

Do you recognise any of the following sneaky thoughts popping into your mind?

- *I am bad if I feel anxious/angry/sad/scared*
- *I'm bad to be so emotional*
- *The way I react emotionally is a sign of weakness*
- *If I was a normal person I would be happy and upbeat all the time*
- *If I am anxious, no one will like being around me*

Activity

Now let's put these in order.

Ranking your thoughts and beliefs

Out of the above unconscious thoughts and beliefs you have, take the top 5 and list them in the following numbered blanks (1-5). Once you finish this exercise, let's move on to Step 4 and the next stage of the Cognitive Behavioral Approach. "Challenging Your Self-Talk."

Top Five Beliefs:

1. _____
_____

2. _____
   _____
3. _____
   _____
4. _____
   _____
5. _____
   _____

You will pick this up again in a couple of chapters. Mark this page to make it easy to return to, please. And now on to the next step where you will turn your thought patterns on their heads!

Chapter 4 – Step 4. Learn the Thinking Styles Which Make You Most Anxious and Turn Them Around

We have been looking at thoughts and beliefs you have about yourself, other people and the world or life. Now we are going to dive in a bit deeper and explore the WAY you think. I expect that we will find a few thinking styles you use every day which tend to aggravate your anxiety.

STYLES OF THINKING

Just to put this in context and keep that steady beam of compassion for yourself going it is will help you to understand why we all have these thinking patterns – we all have them. It isn't only you!

People are very amazing things. We are tender and tough, complex and simple, ingenious and naïve…. And that is just in any one minute! One of the things we do really well is 'trying to protect ourselves.' We are aware of our tendency to feel hurt and get anxious depending what is happening. Then we gradually build up a style of thinking that is an attempt to protect ourselves from the possible pain of being caught out, being exposed, having our worst fears happen and all the other 'awfulizing' things we tuck away inside ourselves.

Here are some very typical examples. I can tell you now that EVERYONE (including myself) has variations of these thinking styles so don't worry if you recognise these in yourself. These are just you being human. And it is you trying to protect yourself from more pain. However what you haven't caught up with yet is that these styles don't help any more – at one point in your life they did – but not now. However, the Great thing about being a human is that you can change these thought patterns when you recognise that they are not helping you get out of that Vicious Cycle of thoughts – feelings – behaviour – body state - thoughts about that – feelings about that – behaviour about that ….and on and on….

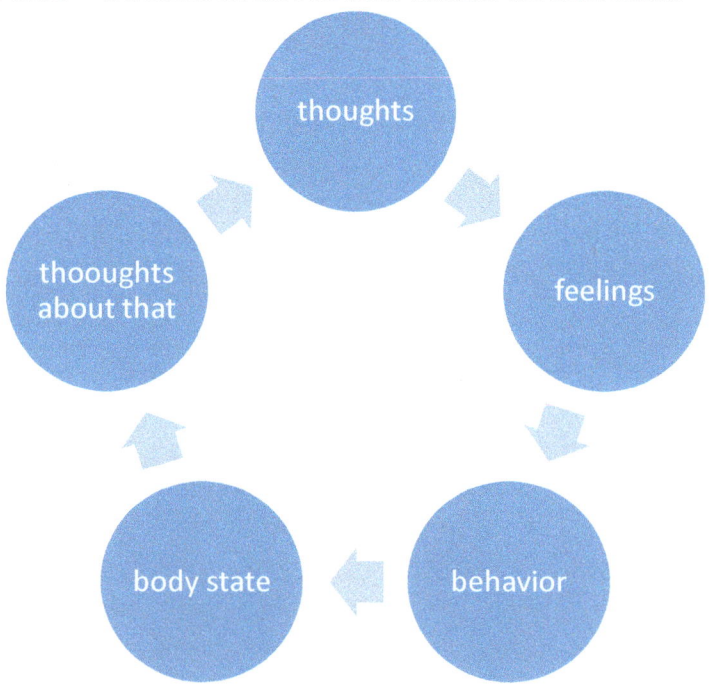

So, let'shave a look at the most common types of Unhelpful Thinking Patterns you are using right now.

Putting up a Filter

This style is recognisable because it is so fixed on one side of a situation. In fact, you may often ignore any other point that might give a different meaning entirely.

A client of mine who had had her work praised for its neatness and then later was asked if she could hand in the next set of minutes quickly only heard the criticism – understanding from it that she was too slow. She completely forgot that her boss had appreciated the accuracy and appearance of her work. Or that there was a rush on in the office because of a big order which was why they needed the minutes quickly. So she went home depressed, but really it was nothing to do with her!

Everyone has their own particular filter. Depending what kind of background you have had you will be sensitive to certain types of situations. For example, being let down, being made a fool of. Others scan every situation for any negativity or criticism. They will do that even if the situation is really relxed and informal.

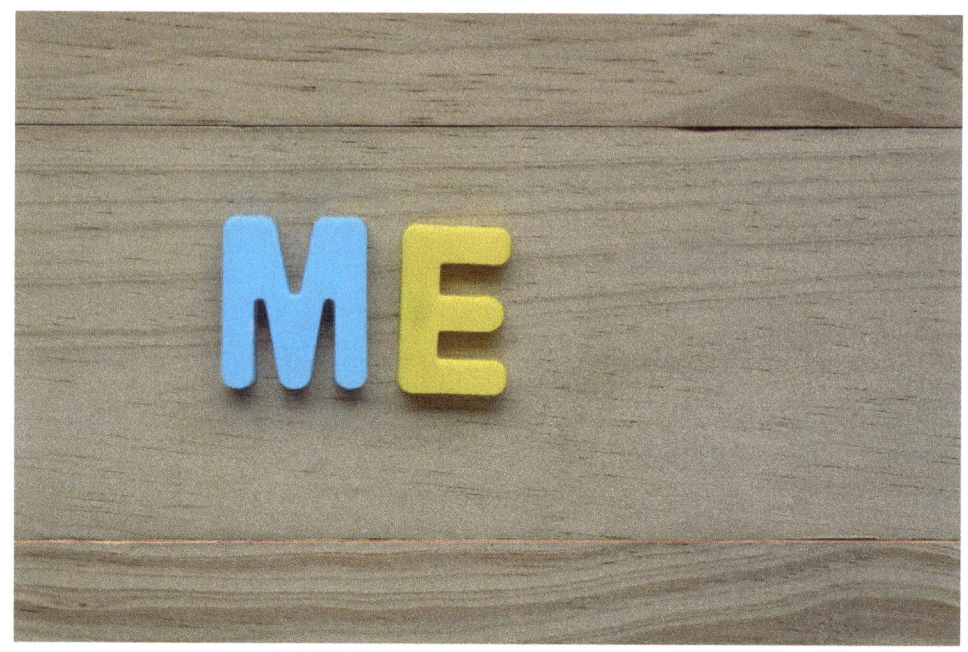

This way of thinking also does unhelpful things with your memory. It makes you very selective. So that depending what has happened to you that hurt or made you suffer before is what you will 'scan' for in a new situation. You may well not remember anything other than these 'hurtful times.' Although, in fact, it is extremely unlikely that other good things have never happened to you. As a result, you constantly expect the same events to happen again and keep re-experiencing things that trigger off your anxiety.

When you put up your filter, taking out the nice aspects of the situation and only focusing on the bit that has the potential to hurt you, you "awfulize" your thoughts. By isolating all the rotten things that have happened to you and making no balance with the good things, any situation becomes a terrible one. In the end all you can think of is how you feel so angry, let down and hurt. The more you think of them the more exaggerated everything becomes.

Keywords for this kind of filtering are words like "awful…it's terrible…… I'm disgusted.." and so on. A typical phrase is "I can't cope with this."

CBT Activity

Do you tend to use those words or similar ones quite often? If you do, it's a hint that you can begin to change your vocabulary. By doing that, you will start to break down the thought pattern.

Black and White Thinking

What stands out about this style is that there are only two big choices:

You tend to make things either all good, or all bad; all black or all white. The possibility of there being some gray in the situation isn't one you allow for. Things are wonderful or horrible. This means that your emotions will often swing to extremes.

What is unpleasant for you about having this style of thinking is just how harshly you will judge yourself. If you aren't the most brilliant, you must be a fool. (remember back to the last chapter where we looked at your beliefs about how you needed to be to be acceptable – speedy, perfect, pleasing, etc.). You don't give yourself any room for being human, average, a mixture of things… The inner voice says it is either a mistake and mediocre or wonderful and perfectly done.

Another client of mine who was driving to work told himself he was stupid when took the wrong off ramp and had to drive several miles round about to get back on the right track again. One easily made mistake, and he beat himself up unmercifully. He gave himself no compassion for having had a sleepless night with a sick child and having his mind already busy with the things he had to do during the day when he needed to get home to help his partner with their child.

He saw himself as a weak, useless person, felt ashamed of himself and criticized himself all day when he was talking to his co-workers when he got to work. He spent the rest of the day in an anxious state in case he did something else stupid.

If It Applied Once, It Will Apply to Everything

Because something happened once, you think it will happen just like that over and over again. One typo in your document that you missed because you were busy means "I'll never be able to put out a perfect document." One party being held to which you didn't get an invitation means "Nobody will ever invite me to a party again." If you got sick on a plane once, you'll never fly again. If you got dizzy on an elevator, you will never go on one again. One time your husband went away on a business trip you got really anxious. Now every time he goes away you feel so anxious you are a mess. One bad experience means every time something similar happens you repeat the original bad experience.

The trouble with this style is that it keeps cutting back and restricting what you can do and enjoy.

Another client of mine, who had had a very over protective mother, had internalized all her mother's worries about her and her health and wellbeing. So it only took one incident to completely put her off doing something quite ordinary. She very quickly overgeneralized many things that happened to her. 'My car will break down if I take the fast road home.' 'I'll start to shake if I teach 4B again so I can't take that class this term.' 'I'm always sick if I eat gluten.'

By overgeneralizing you begin to think of the conclusion you originally formed as if it is a Law that governs everything. When you decide that "Nobody cares about me or... I can't trust anyone again..... I would have no friends if people really knew what I am like."

Unhappily the conclusion you came to and stuck with was just based on a couple of experiences and, like the person who said 'don't bother me with the facts' you cut out anything that might disprove the 'Law' you are operating under.

Listen for yourself using words like every, never, all, everybody.

CBT Activity

Do you tend to use those kind of 'all-encompassing words' when you talk?

I Can Read Your Mind

With this sort of thinking style, you tend to make judgements about others, rather than yourself. In fact, you will make snap decisions about the other person and their motives in any situation. "He's afraid of commitment....!" There is not likely to be any solid evidence of these things but to you they 'felt' right. Usually, a mind reader makes guesses about what makes other people tick and how they feel. It's like you have a special intuition that has sussed out the underlying reason for a situation and then you stick to that.

You may also make these leaps of 'understanding' about another person's reasons for acting as they did towards you. For example, "If he sees me in daylight he'll see my terrible skin... She thinks I am really immature. Look at the way she looks at me... They are getting ready to give me a final warning. I can tell" As with all the mind reading assumptions nothing is actually checked out. They come from a bit of intuition, a bit of a hunch and some fear left from one or two past experiences, but they are nevertheless completely believed.

This process of having hunches and guesses and acting as if they are true is called projection. It is based on the fact that you think everyome is the same as you. The way they think, feel and act will be just like you would in a similar situation. Because you think that is how everyone operates you don't really notice to the ways in which they think and act differently. So if you get angry if someone is late for a meeting and doesn't let you know, you will imagine that everyone feels the same way as you. Being so judgemental about other people is a reflection of how judgemental you are of yourself, but it is 'projected' out onto others instead of only targeting yourself.

I had a client who was an extremely sensitive person. She'd been brought up in a house where there were a lot of secrets, and she's learnt to use her sensitivity to pick up any clue she could about what was actually happening. For example, she could sense her father was angry with her mother, but when she asked what was wrong, her parents always denied that there was any anger at all between them. She had learnt to 'trust her intuition' but she didn't also learn to step back and run some other scenarios past her observation to check if her 'intuition' may be off-track this time. She often was right in her judgements, but she was also VERY wrong, spectacularly wrong, on others. This sensitivity and mind reading kept her in a constant state of anxiety as she tried to work out everything that was happening around her by using her hunches.

CBT Activity

Are you one of life's 'intuiters'? How often do you take the time to consciously think of other explanations than the one you jumped to?

Something Terrible Will Happen

If you catastrophize, a small puncture means your car can't be driven, and you will be stuck forever. A headache means you have a tumor on the brain. When you catastrophize everything you often start with the words "What if..." You can even read a newspaper article about someone else who has been in a challenging situation and start to worry that the same will happen to you. "What if there is no medical care available when we go skiing.... What if the plane is hijacked en route. .. What if the company goes bankrupt and I have to leave work... What if my children all turn into alcoholics because they see us drinking?" The list becomes neverending. With a really fertile imagination and there is a catastrophe just waiting to happen everywhere.

CBT Activity

Are you a 'what if-er?' There is a fine line between being cautious enough and being over cautious and catastrophizing. Where do you think the line is and where are you in relation to that line?

They Must Have Meant Me

This is when you think that whatever is happening, or is being said, is really about you. An anxious mother will quickly blame herself if she sees any depression or upset in her child. A newly recruited man thinks every reference to things going wrong in the department is because of his inefficiency.

Keywords to do with personalisation are related to comparisons. What is going on inside is that you are making comparisons with other people: "She plays tennis so much better than me... I'm too dumb to be in this group....She has got five year plans set up for her career, not like me who just falls into one job or another....He feels so deeply while I am dead inside.....They look up to him and listen to every word, but not to me when I give an opinion..." There are so many people around it is easy to make negative comparisons all day long.

CBT Activity

Do you recognize any of these?

You may be using the comparison to make the point that you are 'worthless'. If you do that you will then have to desperately try to find someone else with whom you compare favorably – just to prove that you are not always worthless. It is a very exhausting and anxiety provoking way to live.

Self-esteem doesn't work like that because the point of it is that you are valuable and worthy just because you are you! It has nothing to do with your skills or behavior! Please remember that!

I Should....

Almost everyone uses the laws of the 'shoulds' and 'should nots' to rule their lives! These laws are inarguable, and any change from the rules by you, or anyone else is, 'bad'. Once again judgements come into the picture, and you will tend to be very critical of other people for not doing things 'properly' (according to your rules'). Other people are different, no matter what you would prefer, and they have habits, and opinions that are different to yours. This makes them hard for you to put up with. One man thought his wife should always have a drink ready for him after work. When she didn't do this he felt angry because she wasn't following 'the rules of what was right'.

The kind of words that people use are you should, I should not, you must…it's the right thing to do.

However, you judge yourself just as much and run your life on a set of rules, or 'shoulds.' You believe you have to abide by the 'rules' and that you have no choice about how to act. This is because you haven't stopped to really think through each 'should.' And then as well as irritation you often end up feeling very anxious inside because you are very aware of what you should be doing, but are not.

Here is a list of some 'shoulds' and 'should nots' you might recognise:

- I should give 10% of my salary to charities every month
- I should never be cruel
- I should always be the best partner for him
- I should not panic over everything
- I should be a be quick thinker
- I should never react badly to someone
- I should have been able to predict what would happen that time
- I should always be happy and never bore anyone by being serious

CBT Activity

Note down the 'shoulds' and 'should nots' you use most often - and also note your most familiar thinking styles. If you are not sure, find a loving friend or family member and ask them what they have noticed about the way you think – you can show them the summary below – and think about what they tell you. You don't have to agree with them – but feedback can often be helpful.

SUMMARY

1. **I have put up a filter**. *You filter out any positive aspects in a situation and exaggerate the negative ones that are left.*
2. **Opposite End Thinking** *There is no gray in your black or white world. Things are either good or bad. You are either good or bad or that other person is either good or bad. There is nothing in the middle.*
3. **If it Applied Once, It will Apply to Everything**: *On the basis of one event, you conclude that it will always happen like that.*
4. **I Can Read Your Mind**: *You tend to make up your mind quickly about what is motivating someone to act a certain way. But this is based on some intuition with no real evidence to back that up.*
5. **Something Terrible Will Happen:** *You expect the worst possible outcome and think it will happen to you.*
6. **They Must Have Meant Me:** *You imagine that whatever someone says or does is somehow linked to you as a negative about you.*

7. ***I Should***: *This is another style that operates on rules that must not be broken. You apply these to yourself and others and people who do not follow 'your rules' annoy you, and if you break them, you feel guilty and anxious.*

So now the thing to learn is how to combat these thinking styles and turn them around to patterns that will work much better for you. One again a little reminder here for a compassion break – remember that you have spent years practicing the old style! It won't take years to change, but it will take some practice and time so don't worry if it doesn't happen overnight.

MAKE A RATIONAL COMEBACK AND GIVE YOURSELF 'PERMISSION.'

Listed below are rational alternatives to the unhelpful thinking styles we looked at above. Have fun with these – if you don't agree with any of the suggestions then find one that feels right for you. These really help to break up your habitual thinking patterns and make you reconsider to find another perspective that works better. Remember back to chapter 2 when the chart contained suggestions of 'New Perspectives' you could try. This is the same exercise.

The key comeback (rational) statements for each style are listed opposite the unhelpful style on the right-hand side.

1. **I have a Filter In Place**
Shift your focus
 Let go of magnifying things

For a long time you have been focusing on things from your life that have scared you or hurt you. To stop filtering, you will have to consciously you're your attention to something else. For example, you can place your attention on coping strategies to deal with the problem. Or you can work out if you tend to think in terms of losing something or somebody, or in terms of always being let down by others. Once you recognize what your 'theme' is you can pay more attention to the things and times when that doesn't happen.

So if your theme is about being under threat, focus on things and times in your life when you feel safe. This is you self-soothing!

Magnify: When you are filtering you usually end up magnifying your problems. To combat magnifying, use words like that's great, I love that, how interesting!
In particular, banish the phrases "I can't stand it" and 'I can't cope with this'.

We know that human beings can adjust to and cope with just about anything. Or you can decide that you don't want to deal with it and take steps to stop the situation. You have that right!

Permissions you can use in your inner self-talk: Try changing your self-talk to saying phrases such as "No need to exaggerate" and "I can certainly cope with this."

2. **Black or White Thinking**
    Find middle ground
Think in percentages

The way to combat these extreme ends of black or white is to be more aware of just how different and complicated people really are.

People are very unlikely to be one thing or the other. Either happy or full of joy, good natured or snappy, smart or stupid. They will sometimes be one and at other times the other. They are a bit of each. It is unrealistic to reduce humans to one end of a continuum or the other.

Permissions you can use in your inner self-talk: Use percentages! Think in percentages about the behavior you are using. "Half of me is really frightened and 50% is holding on and managing to cope with this....

about 60% of the time he has no time for anyone else but 40% of the time, he can be really nice. ....

5% of the time I haven't a clue – but most of the time I do well."

3. **If It Applied Once**

Quantify

Where is the evidence for my conclusions?

Overgeneralization is when you exaggerate! It's never just an ordinary small fender bump – it is the worst case of whiplash and thousands to spend on the damage to the car situation! You can turn this one on its head by ignoring those big exciting words like awful or massive. And use words that accurately reflect the extent of what happened.

You can also examine how much evidence you actually have. Usually situations involve just a small mistake, or one or two symptoms which are not enough on their own to warrant a conclusion being made. Throw away your judgement until you have more evidence!

If you overgeneralize, you think in absolutes. You should, therefore, avoid statements and assumptions that require the use of all-encompassing words like all or never. Use words like some, sometimes, a few....

Permissions you can use in your inner self-talk: Use words like may and often. If you hear yourself making a sad prediction for yourself like "No one cares." Immediately think of someone, or your pet, who loves you/loved you. And soothe yourself again.

4. I Can Read Your Mind
Evidence for conclusion?
Check it out

Mind reading means you're making guesses about what is motivating the other person. It is more realistic to believe the person in the first place, or just have no judgement at all until more has happened.

Permissions you can use in your inner self-talk: I enjoy my intuition, and I remember test it by asking and observing before I make a final conclusion.

5. It's Awful
Realistic Odds

Catastrophizing and anxiety often go together. When you notice that you have dreamed up the worst possible scenario make an honest assessment of the situation regarding the percentage chance of it happening. One in a thousand (0.1%)? One in twenty (5%)? Looking at odds helps you to be more realistic about what is frightening you. You can always ask someone else for their opinion about the odds of it happening.

Permissions you can use in your inner self-talk: Hang on there – let me work out the odds on what I've just said.

6. They Must Mean Me
Evidence for conclusion?

Why risk comparisons?
Check it out

If your tendency is to personalize, make it your job to prove if the boss's frown really has to do with you. Check it out. Don't make an assumption until you have more evidence that it is meant to be directed at you. It is also important to abandon the habit of comparing yourself – negatively or positively – with other people. Comparisons are an exciting way of gambling. Sometimes you win and really outshine someone else. But when you lose, you set yourself up for a blow to your self-esteem and maybe the beginning of a long, deep depression

Permissions you can use in your inner self-talk: There is an excellent chance that the person is in a bad mood today for some reason I don't know. I'm choosing to believe that is the reason they said/did what they did until or unless I have evidence to the contrary.

7. I Should, You Should too

    Flexible rules
Flexible values

When you hear the words, should, ought and must- pay attention. This is the moment when you are operating under a Rule and it is time to re-examine all your Rules as you move away from thinking in ways that make you anxious.

You now need to be working out more flexible ways of thinking. Try working out at least three exceptions to any rule.

When other people don't conform to the same rules as you work to you feel annoyed but this is a time to remember just how different people's personal values are. People just aren't all the same.

The way to deal with this is to focus on each individual's uniqueness. Think about the different things he may want. The different limitations she has to what she can cope with. The completely different things they get scared about. Even with people you know very well you are unlikely to know exactly what their values are. You are entitled to your values and rules – but stay open to other different ways.

Permissions you can use in your inner self-talk: People are different. I am starting to enjoy difference instead of thinking that it is bad. I am even enjoying my own differences!

For example:

	Thinking Styles and Beliefs	Permissions
☐	I must do well in everything I put my hand to, and if I don't, it's awful	"doing something well enough is enough."
☐	I must be approved of by all the important people in my life, and if I don't, it's awful	"you can please yourself and approve of yourself too."

☐ I never like people who let me down	"other people always have their own agenda and will think differently to you. Maybe the way they think means they didn't realise what they did was letting you down."
☐ It feels like a disaster when I don't get what I want from other people	"double check how often it really is a disaster. Find a word that describes it really accurately."
☐ Life should be fair	"No one said life had to be fair. It's just would be nice if it was – but it isn't!"
☐ If I'm good, the world (or God, or the universe) should treat me well	"this is like the above life being fair one. There isn't a trade-off to be made between goodness and reward."

Activity

Go back to the section where you worked out the situation in which you wanted to change the way you think and react. Remember it was the one where you took the top example, from your bottom three!

Also go back to your most common beliefs and your familiar thinking Style. Now let's put them together.

Now put that situation to the test. In it what kind of thinking do you exhibit typically; what belief about yourself, other people or the world do you operate on. Why type of thinking style are you trying to protect yourself with that just seems to make things worse?

Now think of a rational comeback for this particular situation and find a 'permission' you can give yourself next time you are in it. Write down here what that permission will be

_____

_____

_____

You have done so well to get to this point and be unpicking your beliefs and feelings from the situations in your life. Do you see how the Vicious Circle works in your life?

You have begun to change that Circle into a Virtuous one by using permissions and comebacks. Keep practicing as they happen in your everyday life and also work through the other examples in your own lists so that you deconstruct your beliefs and thinking for all of them. Then keep practicing. Keep a Thoughts and Beliefs Diary and watch as the intensity of your emotions and harshness of your thinking changes over the days you work on this. It is very exciting!

Remember to be compassionate when it doesn't work out sometimes and you get very anxious. Just keep soothing yourself with all kinds of nice things, make yourself feel safe again. Then start afresh the next day. You're human!

Chapter 5 – Step 5: From Anxious to Assured. The Transformation

All right, let's say you've done it all – you've calmed yourself down, you are giving yourself helpful Permissions regularly, and your anxiety Vicious Cycles have become/are becoming Virtuous Cycles. You've begun to feel much better. What else is there to do?

Have fun, of course.

Take time to see movies, go for walks, go dancing, try new things, attend book clubs, writer's groups, or religious or spiritual services. By intentionally finding activities you find enjoyable you not only soothe yourself – you have fun too. The two activities combined mean that you will be regularly activating hormones related to a sense of well-being like endorphins and serotonin and getting further and further away from having your life run (or ruined) by anxiety and the adrenaline that floods you when you are in that state.

INCREASING YOUR POSITIVE EMOTIONS

As we usually do let's understand your thinking and beliefs about fun before we kick off finding out what fun things you can start to play with. If we miss out this step you may struggle to get into 'enjoyment' and make it harder on yourself.

Activity

UNDERSTANDING FUN

1. Describe your idea of fun_____

___

_____

_____

How did your parents model fun for you?

_____

_____

_____

_____

2. What obstacles are in your way when you think about yourself trying to have some fun (e.g. depression, money, location, creativity)?_____

_____

_____

_____

_____

_____

3. If you have thoughts such as "fun is frivolous," why do you think you hold that belief?_____

_____

_____

_____

4. In what small ways do you think you can integrate some fun into your life?

_____

_____

_____

What did you find out?

When I regularly ran workshops on Building Self-esteem and Combatting Anxiety the most frequent request, I would receive was to run workshops on how to have fun! In particular, people wanted to know how to play freely with their children. It's a very typical 'unhelpful thinking pattern' that grown-ups have to be serious. There is no time for fun with all the responsibilities I have.

The good news is that you now have the tools to hand to deal with any of the thoughts and beliefs about having fun that cropped up as you did that exercise. Pull out your pen again and write down the Permissions you are now going to use and the rational comebacks you can give to that inner voice that shoots your 'fun time' down.

Cheap and Cheerful Fun

Fun and enjoyable things don't have to be elaborate or expensive. Here are some that you can do right away:

- Walk through a park
- Window shopping
- People watching at an airport or mall
  Rent your favourite movie
- Plant a flower or a tree
- Start a garden
- Rearrange the furniture in your home
- Look at photo albums
- Read books and magazines from the library or local bookstores
- Go to a park and lay out a blanket with a friend or a book
- Watch a sunset or a sunrise
- Other_____
  _____

- <u>Let's make it a daily dose of HAPPY</u>

Fun is a fabulous element to bring into your life as you change from being "an amazing human being who lets anxiety run their life to an amazing human being who has learnt not to do this and now has a rich, interesting life, seldom bothered by anxiety.

So let's look at other ways you can bring a different dimension into your life.

DAILY POSITIVE EXPERIENCES

Get into the habit of creating positive, pleasurable experiences in your daily life. One of the downsides to being anxious is that you often are too worried to experience something nice – or you complicate it by also feeling guilty. You are now well on your way to a happy, anxiety-free life so have a go at some of these suggestions and notice which ones float your boat. Then do them some more!

- Take long, hot, luxurious showers or baths
- Have cocoa with whipped cream
- Read
- Meet up with your best friend often
- Keep in touch with old friends on FB even if they aren't local anymore
- Watch a TV sitcom
- Try samples at a deli
- Go to local festivals
- Visit the local market
- Go to local free live music or arts events
- Play a soothing or upbeat CD
- Watch your favourite TV show- several times!
- Tell someone that you love them
- Tell someone you like them
- Tell someone you admire them
- Get your hair cut, styled or highlighted
- Other_____
  _____

CBT Activity

What have you discovered? Make notes about your favourite fun things and your favorite happy things - and make a point of doing them as often as you feel like it. Ask friends for things they like doing as treats for themselves. Try some of their ideas too.

Write down here what you will try this week. In fact, write down what you will do TODAY!

Chapter 6 - Living an Anxiety-Free, Assured Life

Another Step to Try Out If This Feels Right for You

Anxiety is linked to stress so often the things that are useful for coping with stress symptoms are also great for anxiety too. Let's have a look at being Mindful as this is a wonderful way to inoculate yourself from Stress and move away from an anxious state of mind.

BEING MINDFUL: LIVING IN THE NOW

Mindfulness is becoming more aware, more intentional, more engaged in your life and experiences. It's about showing up, stepping up and really being present in your own life. No more living in the past with guilt, no more living in the future with worry and anxiety – and above all no more shame at being the way you have been. It's how we can be more alive in every moment we live. Considering that we only have this one life – that's a pretty important thing to do!

The Skills of Mindfulness

1. **Observe.** Watch your thought pattern as you drift and respond to things around you. No judging, no assuming. Just watching.

Specifically with your emotions:

- Notice the experience of your emotion
- Notice your emotions without getting caught in your emotions. Don't try to add anything in – or take anything out.
- Say to yourself: "I notice that I am feeling joy/sorrow/fear/anxiety."
- Just see what flows past your awareness.
- Be alert as you observe what flows to, round and through you.
- Notice what comes through your senses, all that you smell, touch, hear, say, feel, and taste.

2. **Describe.** Put words in the experience. When a thought or a feeling arises, put words on it, acknowledge it. Don't be worried if this seems strange and unnatural at first. If your emotional role models have taught you to ignore or belittle your emotions, you may be very well practised at being the opposite of attentive and mindful of your own experience.

   You can also try some of the following statements for practice. Over time you will find your own voice. Say in your mind: "A thought 'this is too much for me' has just come to my mind." When you are nervous say, "My stomach muscles are tightening." Describe what is happening, keep it factual as you talk to yourself, call a thought a thought, and call an emotion an emotion. Stay descriptive and keep everything simple.

3. **Participate.** As a practice to repeat over and over, mindfulness helps you be an active part of your own life. Fully enter your experience, but without loving or hating it. Be as fully involved in each moment as you can be,

participating in each moment as it comes, one moment, then another, staying in the *now* if the moment calls for you to be here now. Let yourself worry fully, let go of it fully, observe fully, describe fully - enjoy the process.

Be your experience, completely forgetting yourself. Drift away from the idea of worrying about how other people see you or whether you are doing as well as someone else. Don't focus on concerns about perfection or pleasing other people. Give your full attention to the experience here and now. Think of Olympic athletes, who seem so absorbed with their sport or performance, appearing unaware that the world is watching them. They give themselves fully to what they are doing at that moment, they are in their experience.

Here are a few examples of ways to develop and articulate mindfulness. You will soon develop your own, of course.

When You Feel Happy
- "I notice that I am laughing…I observe that I feel energized."
- "I notice a sensation of strength…I observe that I feel centered."

When You Feel Anxiety
- "I observe that I am experiencing anxiety…I notice the urge to avoid the person I disappointed."
- "I observe the thought that 'I am useless at everything'…I notice the desire to beat myself up."

Activity

Now that you have read over these examples put this book down, sit upright, close your eyes, (after you have done reading these instructions), and take one gentle breath. Observe your current emotions and sensations. What do you notice? Describe what you notice, avoiding judgments about the goodness or badness of what you feel or think. Stay descriptive.

BONUS EXCERCISES:

We will start off this chapter with a meditation whose purpose is to bring you to a greater level awareness as to the nature of who you are. Do the following:

1. *Find a comfortable place to sit, and close your eyes. Try to keep your back as straight as possible while remaining relaxed and comfortable.*
2. *As in the previous exercises, focus on the sensations of your breath, making sure that you are breathing normally.*

3. *It is important that while you are doing this meditation that you put absolutely no effort into what you doing. For most us, we are so conditioned to try to achieve a certain result, or we have expectations of what we should be experiencing. When this happens, we either start doubting ourselves or become frustrated. I want you to completely accept whatever arises in your experience, don't try to change anything. There is no such thing as getting it right or wrong.*

4. *As you observe your breathe, you will experience thoughts, sensations, feelings, and sounds. Let them come and go on their own accord.*

5. *Anytime your mind wanders, gently return it to your breathing.*

6. *As you continue to focus on your breath, you will notice your mind will become more still, more quiet. It is important to note that before reaching this calm, you will*

most likely experience a burst of activity in your mind. Do not get distracted by this as it is natural. If and when this happens, just continue to focus on your breath until your mind calms down.

7. As your continue observing your breath, you will notice that it will take less of our attention to observe it; you will not have to remind yourself to focus on it. This is an indication that you have gone to a deeper level of awareness.

8. Relax your attention and simply observe whatever comes into your awareness. Notice how thought, sensation, emotions, and feelings arise from the depths of your awareness and then fade away. Nothing that you can experience is permanent; all phenomena are transient and in constant flux. Thoughts appear and the fade away. Sensations and emotions change in their level of intensity. Even if you here a sound that is continuous, it will fluctuate in its intensity.

9. Allow yourself to experience everything that comes into the light of your awareness; offer complete acceptance to all of your experiences. Do not at any point of this mediation use your imagination or create a meaning for your experience. Let all of your experiences come and go on their own accord.

10. Notice that you are aware of thought but that you are not thought. You are aware of sensation but that you are not sensation. You experience feelings but you are not feelings. When you have a troubling thought, awareness is not

troubled. You may be feeling peaceful, but awareness is neither peaceful nor disturbed. You are aware of all experience yet awareness is untouched by all of experience.

11. *Who is the one that is aware of experience? Can you reveal the identity of the one that is aware? Search for the one that is aware. Who is this one? You may say "I am the one that is aware," or "consciousness is aware," or "my higher power is aware." To say any of these things requires awareness of them as well. How can these be the source of awareness when awareness is required to know of their existence? In fact, regardless of how you answer this question, there must be awareness of it. Thoughts of "I", "me," "spirit," "soul," or "higher power," are simply that, thoughts. Keep searching, do not give up. Try to find the one that is the source of awareness.*

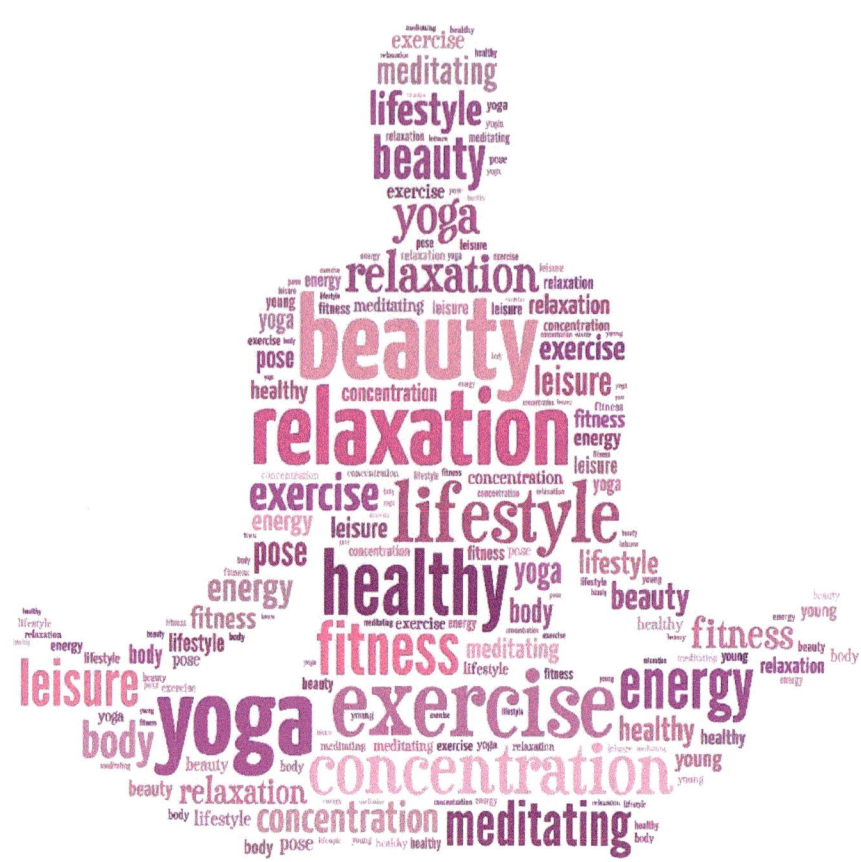

Conclusion

If you enjoyed this book and found something to experiment with, try out, share or commit to we are delighted.

Health and happiness can be found through many avenues and for all of them the journey itself is usually the joy. The destination is what we want to achieve, but it is in getting there that we constantly find out more about ourselves and our own uniqueness. And this is the most fascinating of all.

Until we meet again in another book – be healthy, be happy, be beautiful inside and out.

Sending you lots of love from here,

Maya Faro

For similar books and audiobooks, visit:

www.YourWellnessBooks.com

www.LOAforSuccess.com

****

One more thing, before you go, could you please review this book? It's you I am writing for and your feedback is very important to me. Thank You☺

Maya Faro

More Books Written by Maya Faro

Available in Your Local Amazon Store

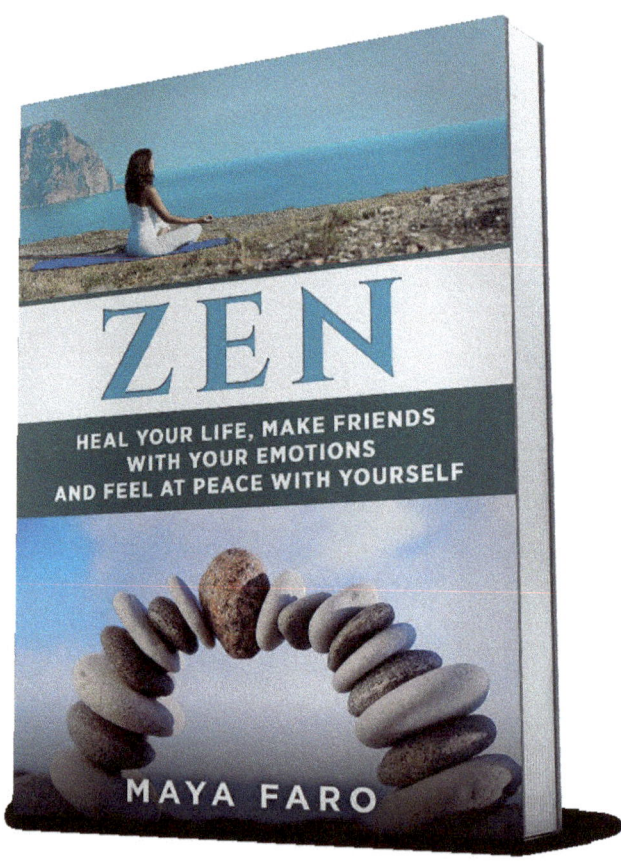

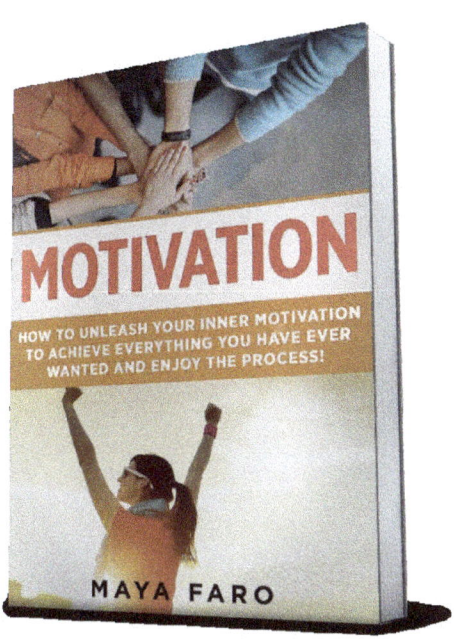

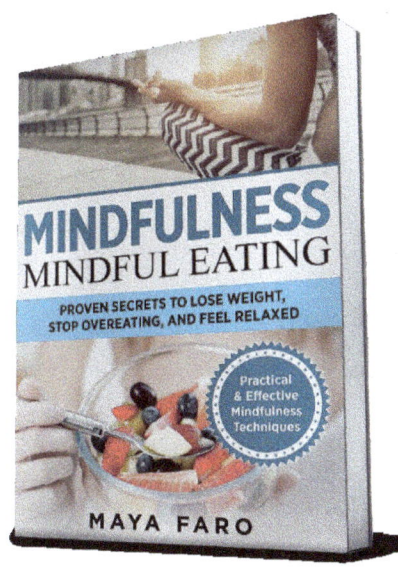

www.ingramcontent.com/pod-product-compliance
Lightning Source LLC
Chambersburg PA
CBHW042119100526
44587CB00025B/4119